When Cancer Escapes The Prostate: Treatments For Advanced Prostate Cancer

Lonnie Boyd

Copyright © 2018 Lonnie Boyd

All rights reserved.

ISBN:**978-1977636652**
ISBN-13:**1977636659**

ABOUT THIS BOOK

<u>When Cancer Escapes the Prostate</u> was written to provide a plain language guide to the basics of dealing with advanced prostate cancer. It is crafted for the average patient who needs to understand what he and his family are dealing with on his cancer journey.

We will discuss common treatments, their successes and failures, and their side effects. This includes exploring the common paths taken as advanced prostate cancer patients move from one treatment to another, when one treatment fails and another begins.

What This Book Is Not

This book does not attempt to be a highly complex explanation of the latest advances and controversies in cancer treatment.

This book is based on my experiences and research as a prostate cancer survivor, and is not intended to address each man's individual situation. What works for me may not work for you.

We will not go into, nor would it be possible to discuss, all the latest treatment fads and the ever changing opinions on them. For those, each man should consult his medical team.

CONTENTS

About this book   i

1   Initial Treatments Sometimes Fail   1

2   The Prostate Strikes Back   9

3   Why Does Prostate Cancer Recur?   13

4   Imaging Tests   17

5   Salvage Surgery and Salvage Radiation   20

6   Take the Testosterone Challenge   25

7   My First Experience With Anti-Androgen Therapy   31

8   Whack-A-Mole Therapy   34

9   The Endgame   37

10   Additional Resources   39

Chapter 1. Initial Treatments Sometimes Fail. Sometimes Diagnosis Is Too Late

When Prostate Cancer remains confined to the prostate, there are several different modes of treatment than can successfully eradicate the cancer. Surgical removal of the prostate is the first choice of many urologists. External radiation of several types, brachytherapy or seeds, and cryotherapy (or freezing the cancer) can all lead to successful cures. Those treatments are not the focus of this book.

Side effects vary by treatment and each patient's particular susceptibility to them, but all of these treatments have very successful track records in eradicating the cancer and its threat to the body.

.

But When Cancer Escapes the Prostate

Unfortunately, once cancer has escaped the prostate, it is unlikely to be cured. It is not possible to put that genie back in the lamp.

The doctors would say the cancer has metastasized, or spread, to places in the body other than its original location. **This can be true if the spread of the cancer was before or after the initial diagnosis and treatment.**

Sometimes initial diagnostic tests will show that prostate cancer has already spread by the time of initial diagnosis. This is usually suspected in cases of very high PSA's. Full body scans often show that the cancer has already spread to the bones or other parts of the body.

On other occasions, patients who have had a seemingly successful initial treatment find that their cancer has recurred. That was my circumstance.

Once a prostate cancer cell, always a prostate cancer cell.

Cancer cells in other parts of the body still are uniquely prostate cancer cells, regardless of where in the body they are found. For example, even if the cancer spread to the liver, it is not liver cancer, it is still prostate cancer. Or if it spreads to the spine, it is still prostate cancer, not bone cancer. This is important, because the cancer cells still can respond to treatments customized to treat prostate cancer.

Fortunately, there are a number of treatments that are usually successful in slowing the cancer's growth. Oncologists have developed a rather successful method of using one treatment for a period of time until the cancer stops responding to it, then switching to another course of action to additionally delay the growth of the cancer cells.

Researchers continue to develop new types of treatment to try when earlier treatments fail. Some patients can move from treatment to treatment for many years. Others quickly run through their options. Unfortunately, not all cancer cells are created equal. Some men's particular strain of cancer may have a resistance to a particular treatment.

PSA (Prostate Specific Antigen)

PSA is used as a primary indicator of advanced prostate cancer. It is a more reliable indicator of advanced cancer than it is in initial cancer diagnosis. This is true whether we are talking about recurrence after surgery, recurrence after radiation, or cancer that has already spread when originally diagnosed.

Definition of PSA

 I now know that PSA stands for Prostate Specific Antigen. This is a protein produced in the prostate which becomes an ingredient in a man's semen. One source I read stated that PSA is what makes semen sticky. While most of the PSA is used in semen production, a certain amount of it ends up in the bloodstream. This is what the PSA blood test measures.

Prostate cancer cells also produce PSA, but all of the PSA they produce ends up in the blood raising the PSA blood level. A high PSA blood level is not definitive for cancer, but it is a sign that more examination may be needed. The PSA level can also be raised by the natural enlarging the prostate as we grow older. An infection in the prostate can also raise the PSA blood level.

PSA After Initial treatment

PSA After surgery

After surgical removal of the prostate the patient's PSA should go to approximately zero. ANY PSA at all is an indicator that cancer had escaped the prostate prior to the surgery.

As long as the PSA stays at low levels it may not be possible for doctors to pin down exactly where in the body the cancer has recurred. Cancer often does not show up on standard imaging tests until it has grown for some time in its new location. This leaves doctors and patients with a few major options.

1. Spot radiation to the prostate bed. Some doctors will do radiation in the area of the body where the prostate was, based on the theory that any spread was likely to be local. This is referred to as salvage radiation.

2. Systemic treatment. Use of testosterone blocking treatment is another common first step. In many cases testosterone "feeds" prostate cancer cells. Blocking testosterone usually slows the growth of the cancer and sometimes puts it into remission.

3. More sophisticated imaging followed by spot radiation. There are some new imaging methods such as Pet Scans which can detect much smaller clusters of cancer cells than traditional tests. Doctors can then target radiation specifically on the hot spots and eradicate them before they have time to

grow.

PSA After Initial Radiation Treatment

Evaluating PSA levels after initial radiation treatment is a more complicated issue than after surgery. Because the prostate is not removed, Some healthy prostate tissue remains and will generate some PSA.

After several months or even years a radiation patient's PA reaches it low point, or nadir. In my case that was a PSA of 0.17. If the PSA then rises 2 points above that nadir, a biochemical recurrence is presumed.

PSA When Cancer Has Spread At Initial Diagnosis

Traditionally, PSA results require additional analysis when the reading comes back higher than 4.0. In cases of advanced prostate cancer, unfortunately, initial PSA often is often in the hundreds. This is a clear sign that the cancer is metastatic; that it has already spread elsewhere in the body. At this point surgery or radiation will almost certainly not be successful.

As treatment continues, the PSA readings are used as a clear indicator of the success of treatments in reducing the amount of cancer in the body. It is possible to virtually eliminate PSA production for a time in many cases.

When the PSA begins climbing again it is a sign that a change in treatment may be needed.

The next chapter will tell a little of my story. Then the rest of the book will detail the treatments I researched and how they work to slow the growth of the cancer, whether the cancer spread is found at initial diagnosis or later. At that point the treatments for both situations are about the same.

CHAPTER 2. THE PROSTATE STRIKES BACK! A LITTLE OF MY STORY

Dealing with prostate cancer is a lot like wrestling a bear. Sometimes you get the bear and sometimes the bear gets you.

I thought I had the prostate cancer bear flat out on the mat and looking defeated. When I was 55 years old, I used radiation to vanquish him. I remained cancer free and was declared cured after five years. Friends and coworkers forgot I ever had cancer.

There did exist a nagging thought in the back of my

mind that cancer could spring up and bite my head off if I ever dared take my eyes off of him. I think this is a common fear of most cancer survivors.

Unfortunately, like the villain in a WWE wrestling match, the cancer bear didn't stay down.

My initial battle with the beast.

I was diagnosed with prostate cancer in 2005 at age 55. The full story of my decision process and initial treatment is discussed in my book H<u>ow To Avoid Prostate Surgery Side Effects: By Choosing Prostate Cancer Seed Therapy (Brachytherapy).</u> Despite anything that has happened since, I still stand by the recommendations in that book.

Considering the state of my prostate at that time (Gleason 6, T2b), my research indicated that the likelihood of a successful cure was about the same with surgery or seeds. However, the initial side effects of surgery were typically much more severe, although radiation side effects often kicked in years later. Recovery from brachytherapy was also much faster and less problematic than recovery from surgery.

Based on this information and my personal situation I chose mono seed therapy, which did avoid impotence and incontinence as i had hoped. (Mono seed therapy, is prostate seeds alone, without accompanying hormone therapy.)

My PSA behaved well for the first seven years after seeding, reaching a nadir (low point) of 0.19 in 2009 and hovering close to there until 2012.

My second encounter with the beast

And then the PSA numbers started climbing slowly and consistently.

At first my Urologist was unconcerned. "You still have your prostate with some healthy tissue, so I expect a certain increase of PSA. You are probably just growing a little more healthy prostate tissue."

But the PSA continued to climb, and by the end of 2013, Dr. H had changed his story. My PSA had achieved the 2 points over nadir milestone he had told me would signify a recurrence.

"Your cancer has returned," he told me, "but I believe it has recurred in the prostate itself. It is slow growing and we probably won't need to do anything about it. "

CHAPTER 3. WHY DOES PROSTATE CANCER RECUR?

Before talking about treatment options when the cancer comes back, it might be helpful to talk about WHY cancer comes back. Was it something the doctor did wrong?

Perhaps, but it is more likely that the doctor gave you and me excellent treatment to the best of their ability.

The most common answer was that the cancer had already sent cells elsewhere in the body before initial treatment. But how likely was that?

A wise man named Partin at Johns Hopkins Medical Center developed a way to predict the answer. He developed what are known as the Partin tables, which predict the likelihood of prostate cancer recurrence. Other researchers have refined and improved these tables in the years since they were developed.

In my case, the Partin tables indicated that there was a 38% chance the cancer had already escaped the prostate before I was ever treated. This was based on the initial PSA, Gleason rating and knowing whether the cancer was on both sides of the prostate.

An aside about gleason scores-

The Gleason score is based on a pathologist's subjective opinion of how much the biopsied sample varies from "normal" prostate tissue. Gleason scores of 6-7 are considered less likely to aggressive; scores of 8-10 are considered very aggressive and likely grow quickly and spread or metastasize. Because this score is crucial in determining the appropriate treatment, it is common for patients to seek a second opinion from another pathologist, hopefully at a "center of excellence." This is especially important if the patient decides to practice active surveillance based on that score, and forgo initial treatment.

There have been lively discussions in the prostate community about whether the less aggressive Gleason 6 cancer cells will spread, or if they even need to be treated. This discussion is of particular interest to me, because my cancer was diagnosed as Gleason 6, but now has apparently spread.

There are two likely explanations for what happened: a) Gleason 6 cancer can metastasize, or b) The pathology report was wrong. Prostate cancer is multi focal; that is there are typically several small tumors in the prostate, and they can be of varying Gleason scores. This is why Gleason scores are often revised after surgery, when the prostate and lymph nodes removed are sent to pathology.

My advice is to take any cancer diagnosis seriously, regardless of what Gleason score is involved.

CHAPTER 4. IMAGING TESTS

Traditional imaging tests to determine the spread of prostate cancer include bone scans and CAT Scans. These are somewhat limited in detecting small metastases. Typically they only are effective if PSA has already risen above 20. Newer imaging tests include a variety of PET Scans and MRI's.

Bone Scan

During a bone scan, the patient has a radioactive substance called a tracer injected into their blood. The tracer settles in the bones of the patient. Then special equipment takes pictures of the entire body.

Areas that absorb more tracer show up as "hot" spots, and indicate rapid growth. This could indicate cancer, or perhaps a fracture or an infection. Sometimes a biopsy of the bone is needed to confirm the presence of cancer.

Once an original scan is completed in order to establish a baseline, doctors can then compare later scans to it to determine if changes have occurred.

Cat Scan

A Computed Tomography CAT (or CT) scan uses x-rays and computers to produce detailed 3 dimensional images of bones, organs and tissues. These images are useful in determining if cancer is growing elsewhere in the body.

According to the American Cancer Society "CT scans can show a tumor's shape size and location. They can even show the blood vessels that feed the tumor."

Pet Scan

A Positron Emission Tomography scan (PET scan) uses special radioactive agents and special cameras to help identify cancer cells that may be missed by other scans. Cancer cells absorb the tracer more quickly than normal cells.

 However PET scans do not show as much detail as CT scans or MRI's because they only show the location of the tracer in the body. Because of this PET scans are often combined with CT Scans.

Other Imaging Tests

New imaging tests, especially involving different radioactive agents are being developed. I recommend looking at the resources I mention in the last chapter if you wish to read about the latest advances in this area.

CHAPTER 5. SALVAGE SURGERY AND SALVAGE RADIATION

On my next visit to Dr H, he referred me to a doctor on staff at KU who specialized in salvage surgery after radiation. I used the time period before the appointment to research salvage options. I discovered a few important facts about salvage options.

You can do salvage surgery after radiation. You can do salvage radiation after surgery. And you can do salvage cryotherapy after either surgery or radiation.

Unfortunately, none of the three approaches results in a likely cure. They may delay the spread and growth of the cancer, however.

.

Why use radiation after surgery?

Common wisdom in the prostate community says that surgery is better than radiation as an initial treatment. This is because "if the cancer comes back after surgery, you can treat it with radiation, but after initial radiation treatment surgery is not possible, due to scar tissue from the radiation. "

Common wisdom is not always correct, even if it is common.

Radiation can be used after surgery, but it is unlikely to provide a cure, because the genie is out of the bottle (the prostate). In fact the bottle was cut out and thrown away. The question is **where** to use the radiation.

It is possible to find hot spots of cancer and reduce them. Another approach is to radiate area where the prostate used to be in hopes that the recurrence is in that general area.

Unfortunately, once the cancer has escaped the prostate it commonly is spread to more places in the body than can be treated with radiation. Remote locations of cancer cells start out too small to be detected by body scanning techniques and only become obvious after growing for some time. Trying to treat all these spots with radiation would be like a radioactive game of wack s mole, which would not cure but would leave radioactive damage spread far and wide.

Radiation after surgery is sometimes used to reduce pain after the cancer has spread to the bones. This process has value but is not curative.

The benefit and risks of surgery after radiation

After initial radiation treatment, either by seeds or external radiation, the patient still has a prostate. If the cancer has recurred in the still growing prostate and has not spread beyond it, salvage surgery would actually cure.

The disadvantages of salvage surgery are the even higher odds of incontinence and impotence compared to either initial surgery or initial radiation. My attempt to avoid these side effects was a major reason I chose seeds to start with.

Referral to a surgeon for salvage surgery

As my PSA continued to slowly rise, Dr H decided to refer me to another doctor at KU who specialized in salvage surgery after radiation.

I found doctor B to be very personable and decided to pursue this option if it would likely be curative. Of course this meant another biopsy.

After a course of antibiotics and an enema, I once again found myself in an examining room with an ultrasound wand and a spring loaded needle gun shoved up my wazoo.

This time I had two nurses staring at my exposed rear while they emptied the samples from the needle gun and reloaded.

Results: the biopsy failed to find cancer still in the prostate. Thus I was spared the salvage surgery, but I had a plethora of further treatments to look forward to.

Chapter 6. Take The Testosterone Challenge

Most of us believe that testosterone, primarily produced in the testicles, is the hormone that most makes a man a man. Unfortunately, most doctors believe that it is also a potent fuel for advanced prostate cancer. Experience treating many thousands of patients with anti-androgen hormone therapy bears this out. Reducing the production of testosterone and DHT(a derivative of testosterone) has consistently resulted in a dramatically reduced PSA, indicating a drop in the growth of prostate cancer.

In many cases, blocking testosterone production reduces tumor size and lessens bone pain. It is not considered a cure for prostate cancer.

Both surgery and medication have been used to accomplish the reduction in testosterone.

Orchiectomy (Surgical Castration)

Orchiectomy is the surgical removal of the testicles. The penis and scrotum are left intact, although the patient's sense of manhood may be shredded. Often artificial testicles are inserted into the scrotum for cosmetic effect or self image issues.

By reducing the body's production of testosterone, this procedure often causes tumors to shrink as well as helping with bone pain. It is not a cure for advanced prostate cancer, and eventually the cancer may become castrate resistant, meaning that it adapts to grow without testosterone. Then there are other types of treatments to try.

A major disadvantage of orchiectomy is that it is permanent. Many men choose instead a medical or chemical hormone blocking, which can allow for a "vacation" from treatment if the cancer goes into remission. This also then allows for a vacation from the side effects.

Side effects from both treatments are similar. They include:

- Loss of libido

- impotence

- Hot Flashes

- Enlarged breasts

- Thinning bones

- Weight gain

Androgen Deprivation Therapy (ADT), or Hormone Therapy,

Hormone therapy, otherwise known as anti-androgen therapy, is used either alone or in combination with other therapies. Hormone therapy alone does not cure prostate cancer, instead it aims to slow its growth.

Androgens are the male hormones testosterone and DHT. They are known to "feed" prostate cancer. Reducing their production slows the growth of the cancer for a time. Androgens are primarily produced in the testicles, with a smaller amount produced in the adrenal glands.

The goal of ADT is to reduce the level of male hormones (or androgens) in the body. The main androgens are testosterone and DHT. Some drugs block the ability of the androgens to reach the cancer cells.

The varied drug treatments are often referred to as chemical castration. They can be used for a limited time or intermittently. Hormone therapy is often used in combination with surgery or radiation.

Common side effects include loss of libido,

impotence, shrinkage of the sexual organs, fatigue, breast enlargement and mental fog.

ADT and Anti-Androgen Drugs

The doctor's arsenal includes androgen deprivation drugs, which block the production of androgens, androgen inhibitors, which block the action of enzyme the body uses to make androgens, and anti-androgen drugs, which keep the body from utilizing the androgens.

- Lupron (generic name leuprolide), and Zoladex (goserelin) and Firmagon (degarelix) are commonly used drugs to block the production of testosterone.

- Xtandi, Zytiga and ketoconazole are commonly used to inhibit the production of enzymes used to produce testosterone and other androgens.

- Casodex and flutamide are used to block the body's use of androgens.

Sometimes drugs from more than one group are used at the same time.

Drugs to treat side effects

Due to the serious side effects hormone therapy can cause, doctors often prescribe additional medications to treat those side effects. Often these are medications to treat hot flashes, bone thinning or depression.

CHAPTER 7.MY FIRST EXPERIENCE WITH ANTI-ANDROGEN THERAPY

In November 2008 my radiation oncologist prescribed a combination of Avodart and ibuprofen to resolve irritation and bleeding in my prostate. I did not realize that Avodart was actually a form of hormone therapy. I just knew that I had pain in my groin and bleeding from my penis that I very much wanted to resolve.

The Avodart (generic dutesteride), had three major effects, two good and one bad.

On the good side, the Avodart eliminated the inflammation in my prostate. As a second bonus, it stimulated hair growth. Aside from its primary purposes, avodart promotes hair growth, much like Rogaine.

On the major bad side, the Avodart pretty much wiped out my libido. Whether I could perform sexually or not, it seldom occurred to me to try.

How Avodart Works

Avodart is often prescribed for men with BPH, or enlarged prostate. Its primary effect is to shrink the prostate. It is a hormone blocking drug, but unlike Lupron and other commonly prescribed anti-androgen drugs, Avodart does not block the production of testosterone. Instead, it blocks the conversion of testosterone to DHT, a more potent form of the male hormone. One result of this treatment is that the prostate shrinks. Which is why it works so well for enlarged prostate.

In addition to resolving my painful urination problems, the change in medication put my PSA back on a downward track. Eventually, it reached a nadir (low point) of 0.17 and fluctuated around that level for several years.

At the five years after treatment mark in October 2010, my PSA was 0.5 and I was declared cancer free.

Chapter 8. "Whack-A-Mole" Therapy

For almost all advanced prostate cancer patients there comes a time when their PSA climbs despite their treatment. It is said at that time that their cancer has become "castrate resistant".

In effect, the doctor has "whacked" down the cancer with one drug, but it then pops back up. So he/she will whack it down again with a different treatment. After another period of time, it pops back up again and a third treatment whacks it down once more. For many men, this process goes on long enough that the patient does not die from the cancer, but eventually passes from one of the other diseases of old age.

Secondary treatments may include a different ADT or anti-androgen drug, chemotherapy, steroids, and a variety of experimental treatments and trials. New treatments continue to be developed, and for many men the whacking goes on indefinitely.

For example, one patient in Inspire.com's advanced prostate cancer forum was treated in 1995 at age 50 with a radical prostatectomy to remove their prostate. Unfortunately their cancer had already escaped the prostate. This was followed with hormone treatment (Lupron and Casodex).

When the cancer returned in 1998 they were treated with external beam radiation. This was followed by three recurrences between 1998 and 2010 each treated with 13 months of Lupron plus Casodex.

 By 2010 hormone blocking no longer worked and treatment progressed to chemotherapy plus Lupron. The patient was then treated with taxodere off and on for six years, until that failed. He then was switched to Zytiga which failed after 11 months. His next step is an immunotherapy clinical trial.

It is beyond the scope of this book to analyze each treatment that was used and proposed. There are many other treatments his doctor did not try. The key point is that with this patient and many others, doctors can keep "whacking the mole" each time prostate cancer pops its head up again. Every treatment had its side effects, some of them debilitating, but it is possible to keep living for a long time.

CHAPTER 9. THE ENDGAME

It has been said that "death comes to all men; but some of us are more aware of when it is at the door." Because of this, each man, especially each man with advanced prostate cancer, needs to develop a strategy for dealing with death and dying.

For many men with advanced cancer, there will come a time when effective treatments can no longer be found. There are a few issues that each of us need to deal with as that time approaches.

- Should I continue to try new treatments to

the end? Will the months each additional treatment add to my life be worth the pain or other side effects I may have to endure?

- Have I prepared my family and my affairs for the time I will no longer be with them?

- Have I reached a point where I would prefer to be as comfortable as possible rather than struggling to an a few more months to my life? Would my quality of life make those extra few months worthwhile?

- Have I made my peace with God and man? Even men who have lived their life with little thought of God and the afterlife often have new new perspective as their cancer advances.

CHAPTER 10.
ADDITIONAL
RESOURCES

The science of treating prostate cancer has dramatically improved in the twelve years since I was diagnosed. There are a number of new tests available that give a better picture of the location and severity of the cancer. MRI guided biopsies and more sophisticated whole body scans are examples.

There have been a number of new treatments developed, some with enticing names such as Cyberknife and Proton Beam.

There has been an explosion in the understanding and use of Active Surveillance (AS). Many men are postponing treatment and its side effects until absolutely necessary.

Researching prostate cancer information and options can be quite confusing. For comprehensive and up to date information consider the following sources.

US TOO International

I recommend Us Too International at http://www.ustoo.org/

Us TOO has an excellent and extensive package of resources concerning advanced prostate cancer available. They will send this to any patient free of charge, although they would appreciate a donation.

They also host a number of excellent discussion forums which can be linked through their website. There are enough men (and women) in the forums that there is always someone who has had a similar experience to you and can share their story, advice and support. Topics include

Treatment Options

Active Surveillance

Managing side effects

Exercise and Nutrition

Wives, Families, Friends and Caregivers

Prostate Cancer and Intimacy

Recurrence/Advanced Disease

Clinical Trials

In addition, Us Too sponsors local support groups in many metropolitan areas.

Finally, Us Too offers a large number of free written resources for prostate cancer patients.

I am referring readers to this group because they are my number one go to source for information of any kind of information and support concerning prostate cancer. I participate in their online forums, have received excellent written material from them, and receive a daily Us Too email.

Live Strong

When I was first diagnosed, I received a great deal of excellent information from the Live Strong organization.. They provide a plethora of resources for patients with any type of cancer, not just prostate cancer. I received a free binder from them designed to keep track of all the test results and other information I received from the doctors. I heartily recommend them. They can be reached at https://livestrong.org/

You Are Not Alone Now

YANA _ You are Not Alone Now is a patient run prostate cancer support site, based in Australia. Their web site contains extensive resources for the newly diagnosed patient. My favorite feature is a unique chart listing hundreds of prostate cancer patients' diagnostic information, type of treatment chosen, and results of treatment. The chart also tracks their progress over the years, including side effects and any recurrence. Entries are made by the patients or their families and contain valuable anecdotal information They can be reached at http://www.yananow.org/

American Cancer Society

The American Cancer Society (ACS) provides a plethora of up to date, easy to read information on their website http://www.cancer.org. They also have local offices around the country to provide service in person, if that is what you prefer.

ABOUT THE AUTHOR

Lonnie Boyd (1949 to present) has written about his 12 year battle with prostate cancer, but that is not all that defines him. Lonnie retired as a regional official in the Social Security Administration after 34 years of service at SSA. He has a special interest in working with and ministering to special needs children and adults, focusing on those on the Autistic Spectrum.

Lonnie has been an active but eclectic Christian for over 40 years. He is interested both in Theology and in active ministry to those around him of all faiths.

He is a graduate of the University of Kansas and a former graduate student at Central Baptist Theological Seminary.

Other Books by Lonnie Boyd

Lonnie Boyd is also the author of the following books, They are available both as e-books and in paperback.

How to Avoid Prostate Surgery Side Effects: By Choosing Prostate Cancer Seed Therapy (Brachytherapy)

This book tells the story of the author's quest to find a treatment that would stop his prostate cancer but avoid the worst side effects. His story is interspersed with a simple and clear explanation of the research he conducted to reach his chosen therapy.

<u>Talking To God About Cancer: Prayers For Patients And Their Loved Ones</u>

A cancer diagnosis for yourself or a loved one stirs up thoughts and concerns that can stun and overwhelm. This book provides prayer starters, scriptures and reflections to help the reader find peace, comfort and strength when facing the challenge of cancer.